The Little Book of Yoga Themes

Anjaney C Handra

Little Book Of Yoga Themes

"The greatest magic is of transmuting the passions"
Buddha

Yoga is such a vast subject, so much information, decades, centuries, maybe millennia of knowledge, from various countries, beliefs, beginnings, covering the body, the mind, and the spirit. It seems like it doesn't matter how long you practise or study it, there is always more to learn. For most people the practise starts with the physical asana practise, working with the body, perhaps developing into breath work, meditation, mindfulness and the pursuit of enlightenment.

Since discovering the ancient art of yoga over 20 years ago, it has been my constant companion. Through ups and downs, trials and tribulations, it has been my rock, my safe place to go. I know if I get stressed, I can find peace, if I get angry, I can burn it off through the asana, and if I am happy, I can delight in the practises.

Whether you are a new teacher, daunted by the prospect of sitting at the front of the class, or have been teaching for a while, and looking for some fresh inspiration, I hope you will find this book useful in lesson planning, perhaps even just to get you thinking in a new direction, generating ideas for classes, and using more of the tools at hand for a yogi, hand mudra's, pranyama practises, bhandas, not just physical asana practise.

Over the years, I have been lucky enough to have had many teachers, mostly unknown, working quietly, diligently, spreading the joy and the mental and physical benefits of yoga. I have studied and read many books and articles on yoga and anatomy, and yet the subject is so vast, thousands of years old, that I will never be done. There is always something new to discover and share.

This Little Book of Yoga themes has 52 themes for yoga practices or themes for classes, one for every week for a year. I have tried to pull together some of the many different aspects of yoga, to form themes for class planning. Some are based on the yogic principles, some on parts of the body, the seasons, the elements or strong emotions. I begin with a few of the physical asanas related to theme, and by adding in breathing practises, hand mudras, bhandas, chants and mantras that work well together, that work on the same concepts, theme or area of the body, start to bring a theme for a lesson together. By adding in some preparatory poses and some finishing off poses, we now have the essence of a themed yoga class.

I have found that a theme, working with a particular lesson in mind that I want to pass on to the students, helps to make the class easier to teach for me, the poses flow into each other better, and seem more unified to the students. It also helps me get back on track if I wander off or lose track, I know what I am trying to teach! The poses are all geared with the same aim in mind, sequenced to direct energy the same way, keep the focus in the same direction, not just a random selection of asana poses.

The best yoga classes, are taught from the heart, from a place of authenticity.

With thanks, love and light
Namaste

The Little Book of Yoga Themes
Anjaney C Handra
Copyright Anjaney C Handra 2018
Published at Smashwords

Teach what is inside you.
Not as it applies to you, to yourself,
but as it applies to the other.

Buddha

Contents

New Year Yoga

After the excesses of the holiday season, gentle nourishing yoga, to begin the body moving again, to slowly awaken awareness and start to shift the energy for the start of a new year, new goals, new challenges.

Prep poses

Easy Pose / Neck Rolls / Shoulder rolls

Up Salute

Crescent side bend

Seated twist

Seated Fold

Staff Pose

Asana

Cat / Cow

Puppy

Downward Dog

Forward Fold

Hindi squat

Sphinx pose

Cool Down

Bridge

Hug Knees

Supported Legs in the air

Mudra

Pran Mudra (Life Mudra)

Mantra

I will practice forgiveness, starting with myself.

Wisdom

"You must be the change you want to see in the world" —
Mahatma Ghandi

Lift The Energy

In the West, when its cold, and wet, its sometimes hard to find the motivation for yoga practice, but once you start moving, then the energy stats to lift. It's a circle, just like life. Move at a pace that feels right for the body, give the heat time to spread. Take a few pauses, stop to feel the energy and heat that is being created.

Prep poses

> Easy Pose
>
> Cat / Cow Pose
>
> Thread the Needle Pose

Asana Poses

> Downward Dog
>
> Plank Pose
>
> Crocodile Pose
>
> Sphinx / Cobra Pose
>
> Up Dog
>
> Locust pose
>
> Bow pose

Cool Down Poses

> Seated Wide forward fold
>
> Seated Revolved Wide fold
>
> Hug Knees

Pranayama

Ujjaya breath

Mantra

Om shri anantaha

Wisdom

*"Energy and wisdom conquer all things" —
Benjamin Franklin*

Detox the body

Using some stronger poses, to create some heat to help to open and twist the body, helping increase circulation, digestion, cleanse and clear any toxins.

Prep poses

Child's Pose

Yoga Mudra Pose (Place fists on outer side of belly)

Baby Boat Pose

Double leg lifts

Bicycle legs

Asana Poses

Gate Pose & Half Circle pose

Chair Pose with a Prayer Hands Twist

Revolved Side Angle Pose

Revolved Triangle Pose

Eagle pose

Locust Pose Variation (Fists on outside of belly)

Cool Down Poses

Constructive Rest

Half Shoulder stand

Reclining Twist

Pranayama

Bellows breath

Mudra

Detoxification Mudra (Place the thumb on each hand on the of the ring finger)

Wisdom

"It is through the body, you realise you are a spark of divinity!"—
B.K.S. Iyengar

Create Space

Without knowing what you need or want, how can you create it? Create the space in your yoga practice to listen to the body, take some time out, pause in the poses, move differently in the poses. Feel the breath, the space, any heat, any sensations, and witness any thoughts, without engaging or reacting to them.

Prep Poses

Reclining easy pose

Reclining leg cradles

Rag doll fold

Tree with Ganesha Mudra

Crescent side bend

Asana Poses

Warrior II

Extended side Angle pose

Triangle pose

Half Moon Pose

Goddess pose

Wide Fold

Downward dog / Plank / Up dog

Pigeon pose

Cool Down Poses

Bridge pose / wheel pose

Head Stand or Shoulder stand

Fish Pose

Corpse Pose

Mudra

Buddhi mudra

Mantra

Ishvara pranidhana

Pranayama

Humming breath

Wisdom

"Our intention creates our reality"—
Wayne Dyer

Clearing Blocks

When we are stressed, or resistant to change, the body tenses and tightens up, pulls in on itself, creating blocks and not allowing the subtle energies to flow. Take a few moments at the start of class to see how the body feels, look for tense or tight areas, shoulders pulled up to the ears, knots in the belly, pain in the neck, or a tightness to the breath. When we feel heat in our Yoga practice, this is energy being created in the body, and we can use this to move and shift the blockages.

Prep Poses

Cat / Cow Pose

Cow face Pose

Chair Pose

Standing Crescent side bend

Pyramid Pose

Asanas Poses

Sun Salutations (Repeat 3, 5, 7 or 9 times)

Eagle Pose

Shoulder stand

Plough Pose

Cool Down Poses

Yoga Mudra / (with hands clasped behind)

Yoga Seal Pose

Cobbler pose

Seated Twist / Seated forward fold

Pranayama

3 part Yogic breath

Mudra

Ksepana mudra

Wisdom

"Breathing deeply and releasing fear will help you get to where you want to be"—
Iyanla Vanzant

Letting go

Holding on to past events or emotions can make the body tense and tight. Focus your intention for your yoga practice to forgiving and moving on, releasing, letting go of any anger, guilt any baggage that you no longer need to carry.

Release any expectations of the pose, do not push or force the body past where it is comfortable, trust in where you will end up in the pose.

Prep Poses

Child's Pose & walking the hands off to each side

Easy pose

Shoulder Rolls with a strap/ Neck rolls

Hero pose

Asana Poses

Mountain Pose with crescent side bend

Pyramid Pose

Back bend at a wall

Crocodile Pose

Half Bow / Half Locust Pose

Tripod head stand

Cool Down Poses

Seated Forward fold

Seated twist

Reclining thigh stretch

Reclining cobbler

Mudra

Apan Mudra

Mantra

Om Shanti

Pranayama

Two to one breath (Exhale twice as long as inhale)

Wisdom

"Life is a balance of holding on and letting go"—
Rumi

Open the Heart

When our heart is heavy and closed, we tend to round in the chest and shoulders, trying to protect the heart by closing in around it. Not only is this very bad posture, it is also constricts the breathe. Feel the difference in the chest and the breath as you practice heart opening poses, drawing the shoulder blades together, and dropping the shoulders down from the ears. Feel the light and energy come back into the heart space.

Prep Poses

Staff pose / upwards table top

Boat pose

Gate Pose

Half Circle pose

Asana Poses

Warrior I

Warrior I with open arms, palms up

Warrior II

Triangle Pose

Dancer Pose

Camel Pose

Cool Down Poses

Sphinx Pose / Cobra Pose / Seal pose

Half lotus / half bow pose

Reclining Cobbler pose with hands overheard

Mudra

Lotus Mudra

Pranyama

Heart Centred breathing (Palms over heart centre)

Wisdom

*"An open heart is an open mind"—
Dalai Lama*

Balance the Hips

The hips are often a theme for yoga classes, and rightly so. As the joints between the top and bottom of the body, they are connected down through the thighs and up through the abdominal and spinal muscles, playing an important role in stabilising the body. We often talk of opening the hips in yoga, with a school of thought that reckons the hips are the dumping ground for frustrations and stresses, it perhaps makes more sense to balance them

Prep Poses

Reclining Bicycle Legs

Reclining leg cradles

Half lotus pose

Hindi Squat

Forward fold (knees soft)

Asana Poses

Downward Dog Pose

Three Legged Dog Pose (open hip)

Resting Pigeon Pose

Extended Big Toe Pose

Tree Pose

Cool Down Poses

Hug / Circle Knees

Happy Baby Pose

Single / Double leg lifts with a Twist

Revolved head to knee pose

Reclining Cobbler Pose

Mudra

Jnana Mudra

Pranayama

Ujjayi

Wisdom

"Take care of your body, it is the only place you have to live"—
Jim Rohn

Find your centre

If the mind is busy, distracted or foggy, and the thoughts are in the past, or busy planning for the future, it can be very difficult to focus and organise the present, and bring the thoughts into a cohesive order. The present is the only time in which we can make any real changes happen!

In your yoga class, give 100% attention, to the poses, keep the breath strong and steady, notice the muscles being used in the poses, and notice how the rest of the body changes to support the working parts, notice the connection through the whole body.

Prep Poses

Baby boat pose

Boat Pose

Double leg lifts

Candle pose

Asana Poses

Hand Knee Balance

Downward Dog Pose

Plank Pose

Side Plank Pose

Warrior III

Crow Pose

Cool Down Poses

Child's Pose

Puppy Pose

Seated Forward Fold

Reclining Crescent side bend

Constructive rest

Mudra

Anjali Mudra (Prayer Hands)

Pranyama

Nadi Shodhana

Wisdom

"Who looks outside, dreams, who looks inside, awakens"—
Carl Jung

Release the Hamstrings

The hamstrings can be tight for a number of reasons, from over working them in other activities, or under working the sitting for long periods of time, bad posture or under active surrounding muscles.

Prep Poses

Seated Forward Fold

Wide seated Fold, over each leg & centre

Easy Pose

Half Lotus pose

Asana Poses

Crescent Lunge

Half Split / Runners stretch

Pyramid Pose

Triangle Pose

Downward dog + 3 leg dog

Wide leg forward fold, over each leg

Cool Down Poses

Reclining Big toe pose (with a strap)

Reclining pigeon pose

Serpent Pose

Reclining Thigh stretch (face down)

Reclining cobbler Pose with arms overhead

Mudra

Pushpaputa Mudra

Pranyama

3 Part breath

Wisdom

*Yoga does not remover us from the reality or
responsibilities of everyday life, but rather places
our feet firmly and resolutely in the
practical ground of experience.   Don't transcend our
lives, we return to the life we left behind in the
hopes of something better.*
Donna Fahri

Spring Yoga

Moving into Spring, the earth and the air is warming up. Nature is coming out of hibernation and back to life. There is a new sense of energy in the air, so bring this to your yoga practice. Linger in the poses for a few breaths, expand the chest in the Warrior Poses, Cobra Pose and Bow Pose.

Prep Poses

Spinal Rolls

Leg lifts

Garland Pose

Revolved Garland pose

Asana Poses

Chair Pose extended arms

Revolved Chair Pose

Warrior I

Reverse Warrior

Tree Pose, with extended arms

Downward Dog Pose

Cobra Pose

Bow Pose

Cool Down Poses

Child's Pose

Dolphin Pose

Corpse Pose

Mudra

Pushan mudra

Mantra

Sat Nam

Pranayama

Kapalabhati Breath

Wisdom

*"Spring is nature's way of saying let's party."—
Robin Williams*

Side Bends

Side bending yoga poses balance the forward and back bending poses, and also help to create length in the spine. They can also open the breathing muscles at the side waist, the deep abdominal muscles, and into the hips and thigh muscles.

Prep Poses

Easy Pose with Crescent Side Bend

Revolved head to knee pose

Child's Pose with Extended Arms reaching each side

Asana Poses

Gate Pose

Half Circle Pose

Mountain Pose with Crescent Side Bend

Extended Side Angle Pose

Triangle Pose

Tree Pose with Crescent arms

Cool Down Poses

Reclining Knee to chest

Reclining Crescent Side Bend

Wide Revolved Head to Knee Pose

Reclining cobbler arms overhead

Mudra

Jnana Mudra

Mantra

I release all things out of my control.

Pranyama

Ujjayi Breath

Wisdom

"Breath is the bridge which connects life to consciousness, which unites your body to your thoughts. Whenever your mind becomes scattered, use your breath as the means to take hold of your mind again. "—
Thich Nhat Hanh

Root Chakra

The Chakras, in the ancient texts, are wheels, the spinning energy centres of the body, moving the energy through the body. Starting from the base of the spine, working up to the crown. These are the major chakras, there are many more smaller energy wheels in the body. When the chakras are balanced, the energy, or prana can flow more freely. The body should feel more balanced and in tune. If the chakras are blocked, or imbalanced, the body may feel uneasy, and out of sorts, in these areas. This is the grounding, root chakra at the base of the spine. It is the foundation, the grounding, the connection to the earth and the source of drawing energy up from the earth. This energy centre represents the most basic human needs for survival, the roots, it provides the stability, the building blocks for the other chakras, and the foundations for all asanas. It is usually associated with the colour red.

Prep Poses

Cobbler Pose with forward fold

Easy Pose with a twist

Staff Pose

Thunderbolt pose

Asana Poses

Hindi squat

Forward Fold (Back of hands to earth)

Hero pose / Reclining Hero pose (on a block)

Low Lunge (back knee down)

Warrior II (focus on the feet grounding down)

Cool Down Poses

Wide leg forward fold

Bridge Pose

Constructive rest

Savasana

Mudra

Muladhara Mudra

Mantra

Ong Namo Guru Dev Namo

Wisdom

"If you have built castles in the air, your work need not be lost; that is where they should be. Now put the foundations under them."—
Henry David Thoreau

Sacral Chakra

Svadhisthana, the second Sacral Chakra, sits at the hips, roughly half way between the navel and the base of the spine. Usually depicted with the colour orange, and being associated with the creativity, relationships. pleasure and energy to fuel change.
Tight hips, might be the bodies way of asking to loosen a tight grip on life, and

Prep Poses

Easy Pose

Seated hip circles

Seated forward fold (soft knees)

Cat / cow pose

Low Lunge

Downward dog, with bent legs, walking feet

Asana Poses

Goddess pose

Warrior II

Reverse Warrior

Runners stretch

Lizard Pose

Frog Pose

Cool Down Poses

Cat / Cow pose (notice any changes in the hips)

Downward dog Pose (notice changes in the hips)

Pigeon pose, with a fold

Happy baby (hold each side for a few breaths)

Bhanda

Uddiyana Bhandha

Mudra

Dhyani Mudra

Pranayama

Kapalabhati

Wisdom

*"The hips don't lie." —
Shakira*

Solar Plexus Chakra

The third chakra, Manipura, is located between the navel and the solar plexus, and is usually associated with the colour yellow. This chakra represents the centre of vitality in the body, the digestive fire, the nourishment for all the bodily functions, and in controlling the body's energy and strength.

Prep Poses

Legs in the air pose (support under tail bone)

Legs in the air pose , lift head and arms, spread

fingers,

Spinal rolls into boat pose / Baby boat pose

Asana Poses

Sun Salutations

Three legged dog pose

Tiger Pose

Chair Pose

Chair pose with a twist

Side Plank

Locust Pose

Bow Pose

Cool Down Poses

Seated twist

Supported legs in the air pose (against a wall)

Reclining twist

Mudra

Matangi mudra

Mantra

I am strong

Pranayama

Kapalabhati

Wisdom

*"The secret of change is to focus all of your energy, not on fighting the old, but on building the new." —
Socrates*

Heart Chakra

The fourth Chakra, Anahata, is related to the heart space, located in the centre of the chest. Usually depicted with the colour green, and a 12 petal lotus. The fourth Chakra, is thought to be the seat of "self", and the chakra governing feelings, emotions, bliss, empathy and kindness.

Prep Poses

Cow face pose

Cobra Pose

Up dog pose

Bridge pose

Asana Poses

Mountain pose / Upward salute / standing back bend

Warrior I, & open arms, fingers spread

Downward dog pose

Wild thing

Dancer pose

Locust pose

camel pose

Crow pose

Cool Down Poses

Seated twist

Yoga mudra

Supported legs in the air / legs against a wall

Mudra

Lotus mudra

Mantra

Yam

Pranayama

Heart breath, place both hand over the heart centre, and focus on the expansion of the chest

Wisdom

"The way is not in the sky. The way is in the heart."—Buddha

Throat Chakra

The fifth chakra, Visuddha, represents the voice of the body, allowing the thoughts to be expressed, and heard, usually depicted in the colour blue. This chakra is also linked to truth and purpose.

Prep Poses

Staff pose

Neck Rolls

Easy neck release

Cat / cow with Lion pose

Reclining Nose to knee

Asana Poses

Puppy pose

Cobra Pose

Knees chest and chin pose

Locust pose

Variation, hands at sides or clasped behind

Shoulder stand

Plough pose

Cool Down Poses

Fish pose

Extended fish pose

Legs in the air pose

Mudra

Shell Mudra

Mantra

I speak my truth

Pranayama

Humming breath

Wisdom

*"No man means all he says, and yet very few say
all they mean, for words are slippery, and thoughts
are viscous."—
Henry Brook Adams*

Third Eye Chakra

The sixth chakra, Ajna, situated roughly between the eyebrows, just above the nose. Belief is that it relates to intuition and foresight, and is usually represented in the colour indigo.

Prep Poses

Easy pose

Cow face pose

Wide leg forward fold

Asana Poses

Pyramid pose

Dolphin pose

Elbow plank

Warrior III

Wide leg fold with a twist

Camel pose

Wheel pose

Cool Down Poses

Child's pose

Prone corpse pose

Yoga nidra

Mudra

Serenity mudra

Mantra

AUM (Om)

Pranayama

Alternate nostril breath

Wisdom

*"Intuition is seeing with the soul"—
Dean Koontz*

Crown chakra

Sahasrara is the seventh chakra, sitting at the crown of the head. It is usually represented in the colour violet, and associated with spirituality.

Prep Poses

Constructive rest

Hug Knees

Spinal rolls

Baby pigeon pose, walking hands to each side

Bridge pose

Asana Poses

Cat /cow pose

Puppy pose

Dolphin pose

Downward dog pose

Tree pose with arms overhead

Shoulder stand or half shoulder stand

Supported head stand (variations)

Cool Down Poses

Child's pose

Yoga Mudra

Half Lotus pose

Corpse pose

Mudra

Crown chakra mudra

Mantra

AH, to release and let go

Pranayama

Skull shining breath or alternate nostril breathing

Wisdom

"Before enlightenment - chop wood, carry water. After enlightenment – chop wood, carry water."—Zen Buddhist Proverb

Tuning up the chakras

Energy needs to move, so we need to ensure we give it the space in the body to move freely. This practise works through the seven major chakras, starting at the roots, the foundations and moving upwards.

Prep Poses

Mountain pose with prayer hands, upward salute,

Crescent arms, lift to balls of feet

Tree Pose

Chair pose,

Chair pose with a twist & prayer hands

Hindi squat

Forward fold

Asana Poses

Downward dog pose, walking feet

Low lunge

Warrior I

 Variations lifted back heel, crescent side bend

Warrior III

Plank pose

Cobra pose

Half bow / half Locust pose

Supported shoulder stand

Fish pose

Cool Down Poses

Supported legs in the air pose

Reclining twist

Corpse pose

Mudra

Prayer hands, Anjali mudra

Pranayama

Ujjayi breath

Wisdom

"Yoga takes you by the scuff of the neck, and takes you on a journey, whether you like it or not"—Vanda Scaravelli

Full Moon Yoga

With each Full moon comes a time to release, to forgive and let go of negative thoughts and emotions. Holding onto to these not only blocks the body's energy, it is also in the space needed for new growth. Move slowly, linger in the poses, especially if it feels "right", or just what is needed at that moment.

Prep Poses

Child's Pose

Thread the needle pose

Yoga mudra

Moving Cat / Cow pose

Asana Poses

Mountain Pose

Crescent Pose

Forward fold, back of hands on earth

Goddess Pose

Warrior II / Bowing Warrior Pose

Triangle pose

Cool Down Poses

Star Pose

Half Moon Pose

Wide forward fold, moving to each side

Hero pose

Yoga mudra

Reclining crescent twist

Mudra

Moon mudra

Mantra

So Ham – I am that

Pranyama

Humming bee breath

Wisdom

*"Aim for the moon, if you miss, you may hit a star"—
W. Clement Stone*

Acceptance

We are constantly bombarded with advertising images, reminding us that we are not slim enough, not wealthy enough, not driving the right car, or living in a big enough house. Even if we achieved all these things, would it make us happy?

Yes, there are always goals, and achievements to drive us forward, but there is a peace to finding acceptance in who you are, and what you can do rather than constantly comparing and competing.

Prep Poses

Constructive rest

Bridge pose

Spinal Rolls

Boat pose

Asana Poses

Sun salutations (x3)

Pyramid Pose

Lizard pose

Dancer Pose

Tree Pose, with crescent arms

Cool Down Poses

Locust pose

Seal pose

Half shoulder stand

Corpse pose

Mantra

Om nam sat.

I m not the mind, I am not the body, I am me.

Pranayama

3 part yogic breath

Wisdom

"Do what you can, with what you have, where you are."—
Theodore Roosevelt

New moon yoga

With each New Moon, comes renewed energy, a time for a new start, to make new wishes, and set intentions for the coming month. Spend some time in meditation, reflection, and come up with a few goals for yourself for the coming month.

Prep Poses

Mountain pose with upward salute

Crescent Arms

Standing back bend

Forward fold

Asana Poses

Low lunge with upward salute

Low lunge & reverse prayer hands

Goddess Pose

Side Lunge(Baby Goddess Pose)

Puppy pose

Downward dog pose

Child's pose /Thread the needle pose

Camel Pose

Cool Down Poses

Cat / cow pose

Happy baby

Bridge pose

Shoulder stand

Fish pose

Knee to chest

Reclining cobbler pose

Mantra

Soham, I am that.

Pranayama

Single nostril breath

Wisdom

"New beginnings are often disguised as painful endings"—
Lao Tzu

Summer Yoga

When the air and body are warmer, we can work with releasing heat, frustrations and stresses from the body. Work with a less is more attitude, focusing on the exhale, the back body, and lingering in the poses. Taking time to have fun and enjoy the practice.

Prep Poses

Child's pose

Cat /cow pose

Sphinx pose

Asana Poses

Mountain pose with crescent side bend

Flat back / Fold

Chair pose / chair pose with a twist

Sun salutations (slowly, holding the poses)

Repeat 1,3, 5 7, or 9 sets

Cool Down Poses

Leg lifts / Double leg lifts

Reclining thigh stretch (with a strap)

Half shoulder stand / shoulder stand

Fish pose (extended legs)

Moving revolved reclining twist

Corpse pose

Mudra

Anjali mudra

Mantra

Let it go

Pranayama

Full yogic breath

Wisdom

"Where your attention goes, energy flows"—
James Redfield

Learn to Listen

Take some time in your yoga practice, to pause in the poses, to listen to the breath, to listen to the whispers in the body, the subtle messages it is sending you. Your body is a truly amazing creation, it can grow, strengthen and heal itself. It knows exactly what it needs, water, food, rest, you just need to find that silence to learn to listen.

Prep Poses

Easy pose (eyes closed)

Neck rolls

Shoulder rolls

Hip circles

Cow face arms

Asana Poses

Hindi squat

Forward Fold

Pyramid pose

Low lunge

Reverse side angle pose

Reverse triangle pose

Half locust / half bow pose

Cool Down Poses

Child's pose

Legs in the air against a wall

Variation (add a bolster under hips)

Prone savanasa (hold elbows, rest head)

Mudra

Gyan Mudra

Pranyama

Ujjayi breath

Wisdom

"Your body exists in the past, your mind exists in the future. .In yoga they come together"—
B.K.S Iyengar

Igniting the fire

Feeling the heat in the yoga poses, warms the body and brings awareness the creation of energy. A strong core practise can create the energy needed for life, for healing, or for change. Work with the attention on Uddiyana bandha, the root lock, pulling the abdomen in and up, pulling in across the abdomen and pulling up the pelvic floor muscles on th exhale. This zipping up, and belting in action across the abdomen gives a stability to the back and intensity to the poses.

Prep Poses

Legs in the air, lift head and arms

Double leg lifts

Scissor pose

Baby boat pose

Boat pose & balancing boat pose

Hand knee balance pose

Asana Poses

Rag doll fold

Flat back (variations arms at sides, arms extended)

Downward dog

Warrior I

Warrior III

Crow Pose

Cool Down Poses

Yoga mudra pose, fists in belly and fold

Bridge pose

Half shoulder stand /Shoulder stand

Mudra

Kali Mudra

Mantra

Om Namah Shivaya

Pranayama

Breath of fire

Wisdom

"That which does not kill us, makes us stronger"
—Friederich Nietzche

Finding Balance

It is a constant struggle to find balance in life, in the internal and external forces, the Ying and the Yang energy and the constant change and motion of time. Finding balance is a lifetimes work.

In balancing Yoga poses, find a point to gaze at, just in front or on the horizon, a Drishti point and softly settle the gaze, the focus here. Keep a busy mind focusing on one thing, the Drishti point, as you take the body into the balancing poses.

Prep Poses

Mountain Pose

Forward Fold

Flat Back

Hindi Squat

Asana Poses

Crow Pose

Standing knee circles

Shiva Twist

Tree Pose

Five pointed Star Pose

Half Moon Pose

Cool Down Poses

Happy Baby

Reclining Thigh Stretch

Recling leg cradle

Moving Reclining Twist lying on side opening arms

Mudra

Ushas Mudra

Pranayama

Equal Breath

Wisdom

"Yoga allows you to rediscover a sense of wholeness in your life, where you do not feel like you are constantly trying to fit broken pieces together."—B.K.S Iyengar

Twists

Twisting poses rejuvenate the body, moving the blood supply through the organs, and nourishing the spinal cord. Always lengthen the spine before twists, and stay present and focused in the twist. Feel the breath in the space created and feel the breath in the area being compressed. Always balance a twist practice with forward, side and back bends.

Prep Poses

Easy Pose with Upward Salute

Easy pose with a Crescent side bend

Easy Pose with a seated twist

Thread the Needle Pose

Mountain pose

Standing baby back bend

Forward Fold

Asana Poses

Crescent Lunge with a Revolved Twist

Chair pose, with Prayer Hands twist

Eagle Pose

Twisted Downward Dog

Cool Down Poses

Child's Pose

Moving Seal Pose

Bridge Pose

Reclining Twist bent Knees

Reclining Twist Straight Legs

Mudra

Tattva Mudra

Pranayama

Kapalabhati Breath

Wisdom

"There is nothing permanent except change."
—Heraclutis

Forward Bends

Forward bends stretch the back of the body, the legs the torso and lengthen the spine. They can also be a good time to close the eyes and turn the attention inwards, noticing more acutely the breath, the internal sensations and the chatter of the mind. Keep the spine and neck long and extended in forward bends, always finding length, and resisting the urge to curl into the pose.

Balance a forward bending practice, with side and back bends and a twist.

Prep Poses

Seated Forward Fold / Seated Head to knee pose

Seated Wide fold

Seated Revolved Wide Fold

Asana Poses

Forward Fold Holding Elbows

Forward Fold Holding Ankles

Forward Fold hands under soles feet

Standing Big Toe Pose, head to knee

Pyramid Pose

Downward Dog

Pigeon Pose & fold

Cool Down Poses

Standing Wide fold hands to earth

Standing Wide Fold Hands to ankle, nose to knee

Seated Twist

Cobbler pose & fold

Mudra

Yoga Mudra

Pranyama

Ujjayi Breath

Wisdom

"I want the world to realise that turning inwards is the greatest joy. In comparison, any other pleasure is a regressive step."—
Sadhguru

Release the tension - Shoulders

The neck and shoulders can be one of the areas that stress gathers. Notice that when you are stressed or tense your shoulders pull up towards the ears, and when you breathe and relax they naturally fall back down. When you are cold, you round in the shoulders in and constrict the chest. Throughout the practise, pay attention to the shoulders, and the shoulder blades, and think openness.

Prep Poses

Cobbler pose & neck and shoulder rolls

Cobbler pose & eagle arms

Easy pose with shoulder circles with a strap

Cow face pose

Thread the needle pose

Puppy pose

Asana Poses

Downward dog pose

Eagle pose

Dancer pose

Plank pose

Upward dog pose

Handstand (or variations against a wall)

Cool Down Poses

Gentle bridge, inhaling arms overhead

Side lying reclining twist, opening shoulders

Reclining cobbler with arms overhead

Mudra

Vaya Mudra

Mantra

I give myself permission to release what no longer serves me.

Pranayama

Two to one breath (Longer exhale)

Wisdom

"These mountains that you carry, you were only supposed to climb"
Najwa Zebian

Release the tension – Hips

It is thought in some circles, that the area around the hips is the dumping ground for the body's frustrations, tensions and stresses. And with so many people living sedentary lives, sitting or long periods of time, its not surprising the he hips get tight!

Prep poses

Reclining pelvic tilts / low or supported bridge

Animal resting pose (walk the arms around)

Hindi squat

Forward fold

Seated twist

Asana Poses

Long lunge

Warrior I (with lifted back heel) / Cresent side bend

Lizard pose

Frog pose

Downward dog / three leg dog / open hip

Tree pose

Dancer pose

Cool down poses

Hug knees

Happy baby

Windscreen wiper knees

Reclining cobbler

Mudra

Merudanda mudra

Mantra

Om namah shivia

Pranayama

Diaphragmatic breathing

Wisdom

The secret to happiness is letting go
—Buddha

Finding focus

The mind is constantly full of chatter, what happened yesterday, what will happen tomorrow, who said what... It can be very difficult to focus on the present, the only time that matters, the only time that we can make changes..NOW. Put the monkey mind to one side in this practice, use the Drishti point, the soft yogic gaze to focus attention. Keep the attention on doing one thing... the pose. And if you fall or lose balance, do not judge, or criticize or compare, just come back to the pose.

Prep Poses

Thunderbolt pose

Candle pose

Hindi squat

Forward fold

Low lunge / side lunge

Asana Poses

Shiva twist

Tree pose

Big toe pose

Dancer pose

Warrior I (variations open heart, bowing)

Warrior III

Cool Down Poses

Child's pose

Baby pigeon pose (90/90 knees)

Hug knees/Happy baby

Mudra

Ksepana mudra

Mantra

I am here and now.

Pranayama

Cooling breath

Wisdom

"Yoga is not about touching your toes, it is about what you learn on the way down"—
Jigar Gor

Autumn Yoga

Take a leaf out of nature, think of the changing seasons, slow down, start to draw inwards in your yoga practice. Move slowly allowing the body to warm and settle into the poses. Don't hold stationary poses, move in and out of the poses, helping to increase fluidity in the spine and joints.

Prep Poses

Seated forward fold / upwards salute /

Seated side bend /Seated twist

Lotus pose /half lotus

Lion pose

Asana Poses

Sun Salutations

Tree Pose

Warrior II

Ext side angle pose

Triangle pose

Half moon / Sugar cane pose

Wide Forward fold

Cool Down Poses

Child's pose

Sphinx, Cobra & Seal pose

Wide seated forward fold, over each leg

Moving bridge, inhale arms over head

Inversion – headstand / half shoulder stand/
Shoulder stand or legs in the air

Yoga nidra

Mudra

Rudra mudra

Mantra

Om Shanti, shanti, shanti

Pranayama

Viloma breath (pause after inhale, & after exhale)

Wisdom

*"Yoga teaches us to cure what need not be endured,
and endure what cannot be cured"—*
B.K.S Inyegar

Find the Psoas

The Psoas is one of the deep abdominal muscles, connecting legs to torso. The psoas can become weak or tight from today's modern life, often too much sitting! Strengthening the deep core and the back muscles, working into the psoas can hep avoid back and musculoskeletal pain. Try adding mula bandha to further enhance the practice.

Prep Poses

Boat pose (half boat with bent knees)

Hero pose

Camel pose

Variations (heel of hand on back waist/ holding elbows behind)

Asana Poses

Low lunge

Low lunge with upward salute

Low lunge with crescent side bend

One leg plank

Downward dog with walking feet, sway hips

Three leg dog with open hip

Bridge pose (supported with a block)

Variation release the gluteal muscles/ lift heels

Wheel pose

Cool Down Poses

Hug knees

Constructive rest

Windscreen wiper knees

Reclining thigh stretch

Mudra

Prana Mudra

Mantra

I am strong, I am able, I am calm

Pranayama

Ujjayi breath

Wisdom

"You must find the place inside yourself where nothing is impossible"—
Deepak Chopra

Challenges

Sometimes you will have to teach poses that you cannot yet do, or that challenge most of your students. We don't have to be absolutely perfect in these poses, work up to challenging poses, opening and warming the surrounding muscles, use props, straps, bolsters, wheels, to be comfortable and steady, in where ever you may get to in the pose. Bearing in mind, it is just a "practice" after all!

Prep Poses

Lotus pose

Half lotus with Samarvitti (Square) breath

Cobbler pose, with wrist rotations

cobbler pose hip circles, and lion face

Cobra pose / up dog

King pigeon pose

Asana Poses

Eagle pose

Dancer pose (variations, hold with both hands)

Side crow pose / Crow pose

Peacock pose / Firefly pose

Pose dedicated to the sage

Backbends (Scorpion pose,

Inversion (headstand, tripod, handstand)

Cool Down Poses

Hero pose

Fish pose

Reclining twist

Corpse pose / constructive rest

Mudra

Ganesh mudra

Mantra

Om Gam Ganapataye Namaha Sharanam Ganesha

Pranayama

Ujjayi breath

Wisdom

*"Whatever the mind can conceive and believe
the mind can achieve"—
Napoleon Hill*

Feeling the elements – Earth

To best feel the benefits of an Earth practice, take your practice outside, if you can. Focus on the feet, the connection to the earth. Notice when any part of the body touches the earth, especially when hands head and feet are on the Earth. Visualize a connection to the Earth.

Prep Poses

Reclining tree pose / Reclining big toe pose

Child's pose

Hero pose

Squat

Forward fold

Asana Poses

Candle pose

Mountain pose (feel the feet)

Variations roll onto the balls of the feet,

Lift onto the heels and inside /outside

Standing splits

Downward dog pose

Goddess Pose / Elephant pose

Side Lunge

Runners stretch

Cool Down Poses

Seated forward fold

Seated head to knee pose

Constructive rest

Mudra

Pran mudra

Mantra

I breathe in peace, I breathe out peace, I am peace.

A peaceful world begins with me.

Pranayama

Sama Vritti (Equal breath)

Wisdom

"All things must come to he soul from their roots, from where it is planted."—
St. Theresa of Avilla

Feeling the elements – Water

Water is essential for the body. It nourishes, refreshes, lubricates, keeps the body moving fluidly.
It is a associated with a source of creativity, healing, calming, and an adaptability and flow. All useful qualities in our yoga practice.

Prep Poses

Thunderbolt pose with crescent side bend

Thunderbolt pose with twist

Moving cat / cow pose

Table top pose, sway hips, figure 8 movement

Thread the needle pose

Asana Poses

Tiger Pose

Moving cobra pose

Down dog, vinyasa to plank & cobra

Warrior I, circle arm movement

Down dog moving into pigeon pose

Frog pose, gently moving with the breath

Cool Down Poses

Animal relaxation pose (baby pigeon)

Happy baby pose

Moving gentle pelvic tilts into gentle moving bridge

Mudra

Varuna mudra

Mantra

Mam

Pranayama

Sithali Breath (Cooling breath)

Wisdom

"It is easy to believe that we are each waves and forget that we are also the ocean"—
Jon J Muth

Feeling the elements – Fire

The fire element is associated with digestive fire in the belly. This could be the energy needed to change, create, focus or get something started. These poses will generate heat in the body, take a long relaxtion to let the energy settle through the body, and some quiet time for the mind.

Prep Poses

Bridge pose

Hero Pose

Thread the needle pose

Low lunge

Asana Poses

Sun salutations

Sunbird pose

Ext. side angle pose

3 legged dog

Tiger pose

Cool Down Poses

Sphinx / Cobra or Bow Pose

Head to knee forward bend

Seated twist

Relaxation

Mudra

Agni Mudra

Mantra

Gayatri mantra

Pranayama

Breath of fire

Wisdom

"Why should you practice Yoga? To kindle the divine fire within yourself. Everyone has a dormant spark of divinity in him which has to be fanned into flame."—B. K. S. Iyengar

Feeling the elements - Air

This element is associated with the heart and lungs. Think of allowing the body to move more freely, balance, open the body to allow for more air, oxygen, prana in to the body, and a feeling of openness in the heart and lungs. A breath of fresh air!

Prep Poses

Supine Knee circles

Pelvic tilts

Cat / cow pose

Sphinx or cobra pose

Asana Poses

Dancer pose

Warrior III

Locust pose clasp hands behind

Bow pose

Camel pose

Cool Down Poses

Supine knee hug

Happy baby pose

Supported legs in the air pose

Reclining twist

Reclining cobbler, arms overhead

Mudra

Gyan mudra

Mantra

Yam

Pranayama

Square breathing

Wisdom

*"Still, like air I rise"—
Maya Angelou*

Lengthen the spine

The spine not only provides structural support to keep the body upright, but also protects the spinal cord, the nerve roots, some internal organs and enables flexible movement. Pretty important! Yoga postures that bend and twist, flex and extend the spine can help to keep the spine "fluid", the vertebrae lubricated, spacious, strong and healthy!

Prep Poses

Mountain pose / Upwards Salute / Crescent side bend

Chair pose & twist

Flat back extension

Forward Fold

Asana Poses

Downward dog

Plank pose

Cobra / up dog

Big toe pose

Eagle pose

Locust Pose

Scorpion pose / Tripod headstand / Shoulder stand

Cool Down Poses

Child's pose

Seated twist

Bridge pose

Reclining twist

Mudra

Meru danda

Mantra

So Ham

Pranayama

Spinal breath

Wisdom

"Elongation and extension can only occur when the pushing and pulling stop."
Vanda Scaravell

The Three R's

Relax, restore and recharge! There are numerous times in life when our bodies need to be nurtured, through stressful times, changes, illness or just changes. Adopting a restorative yoga practice, using bolsters, blocks, blankets and straps to take some of the "work" out of the poses, coupled with extra sleep and good nutrition, will help through these stressful times. Think about staying a while in the poses, closing the eyes, really feeling the effects in the body, letting the body be fully rested on the mat, use a blanket if necessary to keep warm in the resting poses. Take long, deep breaths, exaggerate and lengthen the exhale, and enjoy a long relaxation, or a guided yoga nidra.

Prep Poses

Constructive rest

Hug knees

Thigh stretch with a strap

Asana Poses

Child's pose (bolster/ blanket under knees)

Puppy pose

Wide seated fold over each leg

Variations(bolster for belly resting on thigh)

Sphinx pose

Seal Pose

Cool Down Poses

Supported low bridge pose (block / bolster)

Supported fish pose (under shoulder blades)

Reclining twist (Blanket / block to support)

Reclining cobbler (bolster / block under knees)

Savasana (Eye mask, blanket)

Yoga nidra

Mudra

Ravi mudra

Mantra

Ong Namo guru dav namo

Pranayama

Adham pranayama

Wisdom

"The quieter you become the more you are able to heal"—
Rumi

Sunrise Yoga

Traditionally yoga was practised at sunrise, preparing the body for the day, and preparing the body for sleep. The morning practises are to move and energise, paying respect to the sun, and giving thanks for a new day.

Prep Poses

Mountain pose

Upward salute

Crescent bend

Flat back

Standing Cat /cow

Asana Poses

Sun salutations

Dancer pose

Big toe pose

Goddess Pose

Crow pose

Cool Down Poses

Pigeon pose

Half lord of the fishes pose

Half lotus / Lotus pose

Seated meditation

Mudra

Vira Mudra

Mantra

Gayatri mantra

"Tat savitur varenyam bhargo devasya dhimahi
dhiyo yo nah prachodayat"

Pranyama

Sheetali pranayama (cooling breath)

Wisdom

"With a new day, comes strength and new thought"
—Eleanor Roosevelt

Sunset yoga

Yoga at sunset prepares the body for sleep, letting go of the stresses and strains of the day, slowing down and returning inside. Close the eyes and linger in the poses, moving and adapting each pose til the body feels "right", steady and comfortable in each pose, and then come to the breath.

Prep poses

Easy pose

Seated Hip circles

Lion face pose

Shoulder / neck rolls

Asana poses

Moon salutations

Wide standing forward fold

Big toe pose / Extended

Half moon pose

Cool down poses

Seated fold

Seated revolved fold

Seated twist

Hug knees

Supported legs in the air

Seated candle mediation

Pranayama

Humming bee breath

Mudra

Lotus mudra

Mantra

I am perfectly imperfect

Wisdom

"At the end of the day, what matters most is santosha : deep, abiding, everlasting contentment"—Sumukhi

Yoga for the legs

The complex muscles and bones in the legs connect the spine and body to the earth, providing support and mobility to the body.

Prep poses

Easy pose & hip circles

Reclining thigh stretch / Reclining pigeon

Hindi squat

Mountain pose

Asana Poses

Pyramid pose

Tree pose

Eagle pose

Big toe pose

Downward dog / Three legged dog

Pigeon pose

Hero pose

Monkey pose (runners stretch or splits)

Cool down poses

Seated forward fold

Hug knees / bicycle knees

Happy baby pose

Legs in the air pose

Mudra

Vajrapradama Mudra

Pranyama

Ujjayi breath

Mantra

I've got this

Wisdom

"All truly great thoughts are conceived while walking"—
Frederich Nietzche

Pushing the edges

Yoga is not about pushing the body into pretzel shapes. or causing pain and tension, but sometimes we need a challenge, perhaps in day to to life or perhaps on the yoga mat? Try more advanced poses, even if you cannot fully achieve them. Listen to the body, it is only a practice, leave the ego behind and only go where it does not hurt.

Prep poses

Spinal rolls

Boat pose / Bridge pose

Cat cow pose

Downward dog

Asana poses

Plank pose / 3 legged plank pose

Handstand / (prep against a wall)

Firefly pose

Wheel pose

Scorpion pose

Tripod / headstand

Cool down poses

Yoga mudra
Fish pose
Seated forward fold
Reclining twist
Savasana

Pranayama

Ujjayi

Mudra

Ganesh mudra

Mantra

Om Gam Ganapataye Namaha Sharanam Ganesha

Wisdom

"The greatest glory in living, lies not in never falling, but in rising every time we fall"
—Nelson Mandela

Go with the flow

Some yoga poses flow nicely from one to the next, whether practiced slowly and mindfully, or slightly more physical faster movement to each breath one movement, this style of yoga can be good to tune in to the body and tune out outside concerns or distractions.

Prep poses

Cat / cow pose

Figure 8 hips

Low plank / puppy pose

Low lunge with Warrior I arms

Sun Warrior / Side angle and circle arm

Asana poses

Downward dog

Lunge

Warrior II

Ext side angle and circle the arm

Triangle pose

Downward dog /Plank/ crocodile/

Up dog/ down dog/ 3 legged dog/

Plank pose with elbow to knee / pigeon pose

Goddess pose

5 pointed star pose

half moon pose

Cool down poses

Wide leg fold

Seal pose, look over each shoulder

Happy baby

Supported legs in the air / Wall

Pranayama

Yogic breath

Mudra

Anjali mudra

Mantra

So ham

Wisdom

"I equate ego with trying to figure everything out instead of going with the flow. That closes your heart and your mind to the person or situation that's right in front of you, and you miss so much."—
Pema Chodron

Back bends

Back bends are not a spinal movement used in normal everyday life. Incorporating back bends into your yoga practice, will not only invigorate and strengthen the back body, they open the front of the body, giving more space for breath and the organs, the lungs, heart and digestive system. Balance a back bending class with front & side bends and twists.

Prep Poses

Cat / cow / Tiger pose

Seated forward fold / revolved fold

Seated twist

Cobra / Plank / Down dog

Asana Poses

Bridge pose

Wheel pose

Cat / Cow, Dog, Camel pose

Moving Cobra., Up dog, Half locust / half bow pose

Bow pose

Scorpion pose

Cool Down Poses

Rag doll fold

Cat /cow pose

Half / Supported shoulder stand

Constructive rest

Mudra

Vajra mudra

Mantra

Yam

Pranayama

Alternative nostril breathing

Wisdom

*"Back bends are to be felt more than expressed.
The other postures can be expressed and then felt.
Like in meditation each person has to feel back
bends.
—B.K.S. Iyengar*

Winter Yoga

As the temperature outside drops, our yoga practice needs to heat up the body, to stimulate the digestive system, and fend off any sluggishness, mental or physical. Winter in nature is time of drawing in, taking time to regroup, renew and prepare for the new life, the energy that will inevitably come with Spring. Think along these lines in your yoga class.

Prep Poses

Head to knee forward bend

Leg lifts

Spinal Rolls

Boat pose

Asana Poses

Sun Salutations

Warrior II

Reverse side angle pose

Reverse Triangle

Big toe pose and variations

Side plank with leg lift

Locust variations

Cool Down Poses

Bridge pose

Tripod headstand

Fish pose

Reclining cobbler pose

Mudra

Linga mudra

Mantra

Aum

Pranayama

Bellows breath

Wisdom

"Adopt the pace of nature, her secret is patience"—
Ralph Waldo Emmerson

Strong and steady

Sthria and sukha, form part of the yoga sutras. They are the principles for a strong and steady practice, from building the foundations, the grounding through the feet, to the breath, and knowing when you have reached your edge.

Teach each pose from the ground, the foundations upwards.

Prep Poses

Mountain pose (root down through the feet)

Tree pose

Pyramid pose

Thunderbolt pose

Hero pose

Asana Poses

Sun bird pose

Tiger pose

Dolphin Pose

Plank pose / Crocodile Pose (knees down)

Downward dog pose

Three leg dog

Three leg plank

Firefly pose / Side crow pose

Cool Down Poses

Child's pose

Thread the needle pose

Prone corpse pose

Mudra

Kali mudra

Mantra

Hari om

Pranayama

Cooling breath

Wisdom

"Yoga is the practice of replacing old patterns with new more appropriate patterns."—
Sri Krishnamacharya

Journey to the self

People find their way to yoga for many different reasons, maybe exercise, or on the recommendations of a physiotherapist, and it begins as a physical thing. For some it may always stay a physical thing, and that's fine, for others it may become a way to calm and centre the mind. To work out the stressed and stains in the body, and make some time to reflect, turn inwards and find some peace.

Prep poses

Constructive rest & yogic breath

Cobbler pose with neck / shoulder rolls

Wide seated forward fold

Animal resting pose

Asana Poses

Forward fold / Twist

Long lunge / Warrior I

Downward dog

Lizard pose

Pigeon pose

Goddess pose / Wide fold

Cool down poses

Hug knees

Happy baby

Reclining thigh stretch

Supported legs in the air

Yoga nidra

Mudra

Ahamkara mudra

Mantra

I am becoming.

Pranayama

Yogic breath

Wisdom

"Yoga is a journey of the self, to the self."—
Bhagavad Gita

Yoga for the digestive system

The yoga asanas, while lengthening the spine, twisting and opening with the breath can help improve a sluggish digestive system.

Prep poses

Thunderbolt pose

Yoga mudra with fist in belly

Puppy pose

Hug knees

Double leg lifts

Spinal rolls

Baby boat pose

Asana poses

Hero pose

Heron pose

Cobra / up dog pose

Downward dog / twisted dog

Triangle / Half moon pose

Locust pose with fists in belly

Half bow / half locust pose

Cool down poses

Legs in the air / Shoulder stand

Plough pose

Reclining twist from lying on side

Mudra

Pushan mudra

Mantra

Om Sri Chandraya Namaha

Pranayama

Bhastrika

Wisdom

"Let food be thy medicine and medicine be thy food.

"—

Attributed to Hippocrates

Santosha

Literally translated as contentment, in where you are now, but accepting that you will move on from there. It is not about achieving the perfect pose, it is more about applying the right amount of effort to get to where we can in the pose, and realize that is enough for now.

Teach students to recognize their limitations, and not to try and force past them just because someone else can. Consider WHY, they would need to? Standing on your head, or touching your toes in itself will not change anything.

Prep poses

Lion pose

Puppy pose

Cat / cow pose

Hindi squat

Forward fold / Standing split

Asana Poses

Log pose

Dancer pose

Aeroplane pose / Warrior III

Downward dog

Three legged dog / Wild thing

Cool down poses

Bridge pose

Half / shoulder stand

Fish pose

Corpse pose

Mudra

Hansi mudra

Mantra

Om Shanti shanti shanti

Pranayama

Alternative nostril breathing

Wisdom

"Peace comes from within. Do not seek it without."—
Buddha

"Tell me and I forget,
Teach me, and I remember
Involve me and I learn"
George Bernard Shaw

Made in the USA
Middletown, DE
14 June 2022

67173575R00066